BEI GRIN MACHT SICH IHR WISSEN BEZAHLT

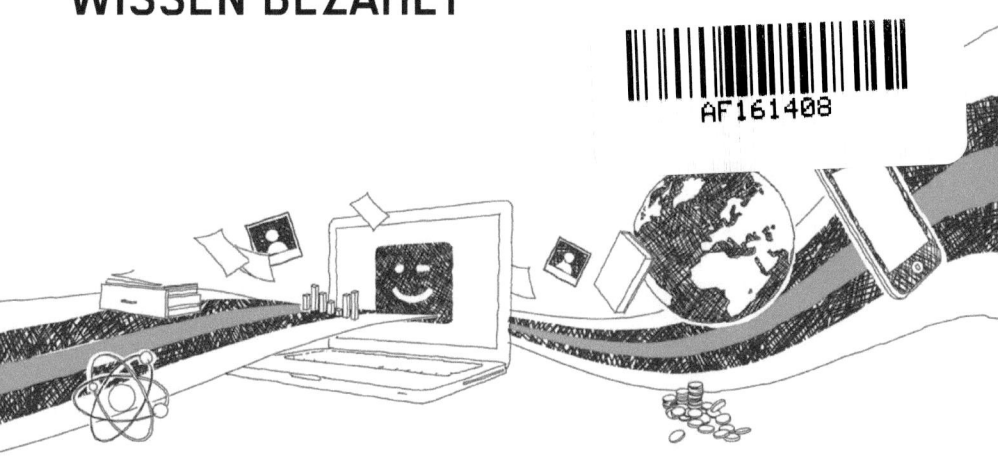

- Wir veröffentlichen Ihre Hausarbeit, Bachelor- und Masterarbeit

- Ihr eigenes eBook und Buch - weltweit in allen wichtigen Shops

- Verdienen Sie an jedem Verkauf

Jetzt bei www.GRIN.com hochladen und kostenlos publizieren

Ginka Tchervenkova

Das Gesundheitssystem Bulgariens

GRIN Verlag

Bibliografische Information der Deutschen Nationalbibliothek:

Die Deutsche Bibliothek verzeichnet diese Publikation in der Deutschen Nationalbibliografie; detaillierte bibliografische Daten sind im Internet über http://dnb.d-nb.de/ abrufbar.

Dieses Werk sowie alle darin enthaltenen einzelnen Beiträge und Abbildungen sind urheberrechtlich geschützt. Jede Verwertung, die nicht ausdrücklich vom Urheberrechtsschutz zugelassen ist, bedarf der vorherigen Zustimmung des Verlages. Das gilt insbesondere für Vervielfältigungen, Bearbeitungen, Übersetzungen, Mikroverfilmungen, Auswertungen durch Datenbanken und für die Einspeicherung und Verarbeitung in elektronische Systeme. Alle Rechte, auch die des auszugsweisen Nachdrucks, der fotomechanischen Wiedergabe (einschließlich Mikrokopie) sowie der Auswertung durch Datenbanken oder ähnliche Einrichtungen, vorbehalten.

Impressum:

Copyright © 2004 GRIN Verlag GmbH
Druck und Bindung: Books on Demand GmbH, Norderstedt Germany
ISBN: 978-3-640-99717-6

Dieses Buch bei GRIN:

http://www.grin.com/de/e-book/47699/das-gesundheitssystem-bulgariens

GRIN - Your knowledge has value

Der GRIN Verlag publiziert seit 1998 wissenschaftliche Arbeiten von Studenten, Hochschullehrern und anderen Akademikern als eBook und gedrucktes Buch. Die Verlagswebsite www.grin.com ist die ideale Plattform zur Veröffentlichung von Hausarbeiten, Abschlussarbeiten, wissenschaftlichen Aufsätzen, Dissertationen und Fachbüchern.

Besuchen Sie uns im Internet:

http://www.grin.com/

http://www.facebook.com/grincom

http://www.twitter.com/grin_com

HAMBURGER UNIVERSITÄT FÜR WIRTSCHAFT UND POLITIK

Fach: **Gesundheitssysteme und Gesundheitspolitik in Europa**

Titel:

Das Gesundheitssystem

Bulgariens

Inhaltsverzeichnis

1. Geschichtlicher Hintergrund... 3
2. Organisationsstruktur des Gesundheitssystems Bulgariens in den Übergangsjahren nach 1989... 5
3. Probleme und Herausforderungen vor dem bulgarischen Gesundheitssystem mit Rücksicht auf seinen bevorstehenden EU-Beitritt in 2007... 9

Benutzte Literatur.. 13

Anhang 1, Organisationsstruktur des Gesundheitssystems Bulgariens......................... 14
Anhang 2, Gesamtausgaben für Gesundheitsleistungen in Europa – gemessen als % vom BIP.. 15
Anhang 3, Ausgaben für Gesundheitsleistungen in Europa – gemessen in USD pro Kopf......... 16
Anhang 4, Anteil der Ärzte und der Krankenschwester in Europa – gemessen pro 1000 Einwohner.. 17
Anhang 5, Anteil des medizinischen Personals in Bulgarien – gemessen als Anteil pro 1000 Einwohner.. 18
Anhang 6, Finanzierung des Gesundheitssystems Bulgariens...................................... 19
Anhang 7, Das Krankenversicherungsgesetz vom 1998... 20

1. Geschichtlicher Hintergrund

Gemeinschaftlich finanziertes Gesundheitswesen wurde in Bulgarien am Ende des 19.Jhs. nach der Befreiung vom 5jahrhundert langen Türkischen Joch zum ersten Mal in der neueren Geschichte des Landes eingeführt. Die dafür notwendigen Gesetze über das Gesundheitswesen wurden zwischen 1879 und 1903 erlassen und in Kraft gesetzt. Die ersten Einrichtungen des Gesundheitssystems wurden auch zu dieser Zeit errichtet. Dazu gehört u.a. auch die vom Staat finanzierte kostenfreie Behandlung für die Armen in den Krankenhäusern. Die während des Russisch-Türkischen Krieges vom 1877-1878 errichteten Lazarette wurden behalten und als reguläre Krankenhäuser weiterentwickelt. Unter den lokal wohnenden Privatärzten wurden vom Staat in allen Orten mit mehr als 4000 Einwohnern Landkreis- und Gemeindeärzte ernannt und angestellt. Auf einer teilweise privaten Basis arbeiteten die in den kleineren Orten tätigen Feldscher. Die bulgarischen ärztlichen und zahnärztlichen Verbände wurden in 1901 gegründet. Unmittelbar danach wurde das erste Gesetz über das öffentliche Gesundheitswesen verabschiedet. Private Gesundheitseinrichtungen wie Krankenhäuser, Sanatorien und Polykliniken wurden errichtet. In 1918 wurde die Medizinische Universität Sofia gegründet, die sich auch als ein Forschungszentrum auf dem medizinischen Bereich etablierte.

Das erste Krankenversicherungsgesetz wurde in 1918 eingeführt. In 1924 wurde das zweite diesbezügliche Gesetz verabschiedet, laut dessen alle Staatsbeamten und Angestellten im öffentlichen und im privaten Sektor gesetzlich pflichtversichert für Krankheitsfälle, Mutterschaft und Pensionierung sein sollten. In 1925 wurde das Krankenversicherungsgesetz für die Fälle der Albeitslosigkeit eingeführt (Quelle: Geschichte des Gesundheitswesens in Bulgarien, http://www.nhif.bg/bg/default.phtml, 07.01.2005). Das so entstandene Krankenversicherungssystem war ähnlich dem Bismarcksche Versicherungssystem.

In 1929 wurde das Volksgesundheitsgesetzt verabschiedet. Ihm zufolge wurde die Verantwortung für die Gesundheitsversorgung vom Staat auf die Gemeinden übertragen. Gesundheitseinrichtungen für Schwangerschaft und Mutterschaft (Geburtklinikern), sowie auch für präventive Untersuchungen und Impfungen wurden gegründet. Ärztliche Praxis in Schulen und weiteren Einrichtungen zur Gesundheitsförderung und Hygiene wurden auch eingeführt. Ein Netz von Familienärzten praktizierte die allgemeine Medizin.

In 1944 wurde das Gesundheitsministerium mit der Aufgabe gegründet, das gesamte Gesundheitssystem Bulgariens zu koordinieren und zu kontrollieren, das inzwischen schon einen gut entwickelten öffentlichen Sektor und einen im Vergleich zu ihm kleineren privaten Sektor umfasste. (Quelle: Koulaksazov et al. 2003: 8-9)

In 1948 begann die kommunistische Administration das existierende System durch den sowjetischen Gesundheitsmodell ‚Semaschko' zu ersetzen. Infolge dessen wurden die privaten Krankenhäuser und Apotheken nationalisiert und der zentralen Staatskontrolle unterstellt. Das Krankenversicherungssystem und die Bulgarische Medizinassoziation wurden abgeschafft. Die Ausbildung in Medizin wurde zentralisiert und dem Gesundheitsministerium unterstellt. Das Angebot an Gesundheitsleistungen wurde aber erweitert, wobei zahlreiche neue Gesundheitszentren, Geburtkliniken und Krankenhäuser in fast allen Dörfern gebaut und eingerichtet wurden. Das Netz der Familienärzte wurde abgeschafft und durch die neu errichteten und zu den Krankenhäusern angehörenden Polykliniken ersetzt. Die primäre Krankenhilfe wurde nach Stadtteilprinzip organisiert, wobei die Patienten gemäß ihrer Anschrift zu einem Arzt in einer bestimmten Poliklinik zugeordnet und angebunden wurden.

Ab 1950 begann das Errichten von Sanitärepidemischen Zentren auf der ganzen Fläche Bulgariens. Als öffentliche Gesundheitseinrichtungen wurde ihnen das Vorbeugen und die Bekämpfung von übertragbaren Krankheiten wie Tuberkulose, Malaria, Typhus, parasitäre Krankheiten zugeordnet. Weitreichende Immunisierungen wurden zu etwas Selbstverständlichem. Ein guter Netz von zahnärztlichen Kliniken und Apotheken wurde entwickelt. Forschungsinstitute und Krankenhauskliniken wurden gegründet in allen Hauptzweigen der Medizin. Als Ergebnis von dieser umfangreichen Weiterentwicklung der Gesundheitseinrichtungen Bulgariens und dem daraus resultierenden verbesserten Zugang zu Gesundheitsdienstleistungen wurde die Sterblichkeit, besonders von Kindern, reduziert und die Lebenserwartung der Bevölkerung erhöht. (Quelle: Koulaksazov et al. 2003: 9)

Die 60er und 70er Jahre wurden durch das Errichten von weiteren zahlreichen neuen Krankenhäuser und Zentren überall in Bulgarien und durch die universitäre Ausbildung von vielen neuen Ärzten in den 5 neuen Medizinischen Fakultäten an weiteren bulgarischen Universitäten gekennzeichnet. In 1973 wurde das Volksfürsorgegesetzt verabschiedet, das die gesetzliche Basis und die Organisationsprinzipien des Gesundheitssystems Bulgariens zugrunde legte.

Als positive Seiten der Entwicklung im Gesundheitswesen während der kommunistischen Zeit können die Folgenden beurteilt werden: die garantierten kostenfreien und für alle Bürger zugänglichen Gesundheitsdienstleistungen, das dichte Netz von Gesundheitseinrichtungen und die sehr gute Versorgung mit Gesundheitsdienstleistungen und –mittel im ganzen Land, das Nehmen im Griff und die Kontrolle der übertragbaren Krankheiten, die Vorsorgeuntersuchungen und die Immunisierungen, das Versorgen des Gesundheitssektors mit ausreichend vielen und hoch qualifizierten Ärzten und weiterem Medizinpersonal, die Ausdehnung der Forschungsarbeit auf dem Bereich der Medizin u.a.

Als negative Seiten des kommunistischen Gesundheitssystems können unter anderem die Folgenden genannt werden: die Unflexibilität des staatlich kontrollierten Gesundheitssystems, die unausreichende Fürsorge für chronische Krankheiten, die Mangel an einer modernen Infrastruktur für Invaliden u.a. Aus volkswirtschaftlicher Sicht wurde des weiteren das so geschaffene breite System von Gesundheitseinrichtungen langfristig finanziell nicht gesichert und erwies sich nicht in der Lage, die Qualität der an die Bürger zu erbringenden Gesundheitsleistungen auf Dauer sicher zu stellen, weder die Letztere in Situationen von Wirtschaftsstagnation und –krise, die sich durch einen wesentlichen finanziellen Überschuss der Nachfrage gegen des Angebots charakterisieren, zu gewährleisten. Als Ergebnis wurden viele Elemente des kommunistischen Gesundheitssystems in den Übergangsjahren nach 1989 abgeschafft, wobei es sich oft um Komponenten und Aspekten des Gesundheitswesens handelte, dessen Funktionieren unentbehrlich und gut war, für die aber in den Bedingungen der schweren Wirtschaftskrise von den 90er Jahre keine finanziellen Mittel mehr zur Verfügung standen.

2. Organisationsstruktur des Gesundheitssystems Bulgariens in den Übergangsjahren nach 1989

Zum einen wesentlichen Teil wurde des Gesundheitssystem Bulgariens in den 90er Jahren weiterhin auf den sowjetischen Modell Semaschko basiert. Das ist dazu zurückzuführen, dass die Reformen eines sehr sensiblen Sektors der Sozialpolitik, welcher das Gesundheitssystem darstellt, in einer jeden Gesellschaft wirtschaftspolitisch sehr schwierig durchzuführen und mit hohen Übergangskosten aus einer sozialen und psychologischer Sicht verbunden sind. Des weiteren stellte die Reform des Gesundheitssystems Bulgariens in den 90er Jahren die dritte Restrukturierung innerhalb eines einzigen Jahrhunderts. Diese Tatsache ihrerseits hat als eine Hauptfolge die Unmöglichkeit zur kontinuierlichen Weiterentwicklung und langfristigen Durchsetzung von Organisationsprinzipen des Sektors, welche Organisationsprinzipen als traditionelle Basis in der Gesundheitspolitik anderer Staaten, denen die nacheinander folgenden geschichtlichen Erschütterungen wie im Fall Bulgarien erspart worden sind, verankert werden und um Stabilität sorgen.

Am Anfang des Übergangs in den frühen 90er Jahren war das Gesundheitssystem in Bulgarien weiterhin auf die öffentliche steuerbasierte Finanzierung hingewiesen. Die Untersuchungen der Patienten und ihre Behandlung wurde primär immer noch durch die Krankenhäuser gewährleistet.

Es bestanden so gut wie fast keine Anreize für die Erbringer der Gesundheitsleistungen, die Effektivität und die Effizienz zu steigern.

Der begonnene allgemeine Übergang von Planwirtschaft zu Marktwirtschaft war aber die Grundlage zu den ersten Änderungen auch im Gesundheitssystem. Diese Änderungen stellten Entwicklungsprozesse zur Konformabilität mit den neuen marktwirtschaftlichen Prinzipien oder aber das Zurückkehren zu alten Organisationsformen dar. Als Beispiel für die ersteren Prozesse kann das Öffnen der ersten privaten ärztlichen Praxis und der ersten privaten Apotheken und für die letzteren dementsprechend das Wiedergründen der Medizinassoziationen gegeben werden. Die dafür erforderliche gesetzliche Basis wurde verabschiedet. Die Verantwortung für eine steigende Anzahl von Gesundheitsleistungen begann vom Staat auf die Gemeinden übertragen zu werden.

Ein viel radikalerer Schritt zur Umstrukturierung des Gesundheitssektors wurde am Ende der 90er Jahre durchgeführt, als das Semaschko-System abgeschafft und durch ein Sozialversicherungssystem ersetzt wurde. Die mit dieser Umstrukturierung verbundenen hohen sozialen Kosten, die nicht zuletzt auf die erneute Einschränkung der sich am Anfang der 90er Jahre durchgesetzten absoluten Wahlfreiheit der Patienten und auf eine sehr hohe finanzielle Belastung der Haushalte zurückzuführen sind, widerspiegelten sich nicht nur in einer stark gesunkenen Popularität der rechten Regierung und dadurch in einem hohen sozialen Druck auf die letztere, sondern auch in eine absteigende Inanspruchnahme von den Dienstleistungen der gesetzlichen Gesundheitsleistungssicherung zugunsten entweder der privaten Gesundheitsleistungserbringer oder aber in einer Großzahl der Fälle zugunsten des bewussten persönlichen Ausschließenseins aus dem Gesundheitssystem und des daraus resultierenden und von der Krisenentwicklung des Landes erzwungenen Eingehens an einem sehr hohen persönlichen Sozialversicherungsrisiko.

Das neu eingeführte Sozialversicherungssystem rief demzufolge ins Leben neue Akteure im Gesundheitssystem Bulgariens. Dies sind die Nationalkrankenkasse (als ein Analog der im deutschen Gesundheitssystem bestehenden Krankenkassen) zum einen und das sogenannte GP-Netz (als ein Analog dem englischen Netz von ‚general practitioners', also von Ärzten der allgemeinen Medizin) zum anderen (siehe Anhang 7, Das Krankenversicherungsgesetz vom 1998). Die Parallele zu den als Vorbild genommenen Organisationsstrukturen aus dem deutschen und dem englischen Gesundheitssystem aber benötigten im Fall des neuen bulgarischen Gesundheitssystems den Hinweis, dass es sich dabei vorwiegend um Übernahme von Grundprinzipien der Organisationsstruktur und der Funktionierungsweise geht, welche aber der bulgarischen Realität angepasst wurden und weiterhin angepasst werden. So beispielsweise besteht im deutschen System eine Vielzahl von Krankenkassen, welche Vielzahl nicht zuletzt darauf hingewiesen sein sollte, den

Wettbewerb zu steigern. Im bulgarischen System ist im Unterschied dazu die Krankenkasse nur eine, dies ist durch das Gesetz für die nationale Krankenkasse geregelt und setzt erneut eine zentralisierte Finanzierungsstruktur voraus, die im Unterschied zum Somaschko-System nicht durch Steuer, sondern durch Beiträge und das Staatsbudget finanziert wird. Das englische System des GP-Netzes ist primär auf die primäre Untersuchung und Hausbesuche einer Großzahl von ‚qualifizierten Krankenschwester' (qualified nurses) basiert, die anders als in Deutschland und in Bulgarien die Vollmächte haben, Arzneien zu verordnen, Rezepte zu schreiben und nur dann den Patienten ihrem obergesetzten Arzt zu schicken, wenn sie der Einsicht sind, dass der Patient eine grundsätzlichere Untersuchung durch den Letzteren bräuchte. Im bulgarischen GP-Netz geht es wiederum nur um Ärzte der allgemeinen Medizin, die sich selbständig gemacht haben und in ihren privaten Praxis sowohl Patienten der nationalen Krankenkasse gegen Zurückerstattung der daraus entstehenden Kosten durch die Krankenkasse und durch einen kleinen und pro Besuch anfallenden vom Patienten dem Arzt zu bezahlenden Barbeitrag behandeln, als auch Privatpatienten, worunter im bulgarischen Kontext keine private Krankenversicherung zu verstehen ist, sondern die 100%-ige Bezahlung in bar für die entstehenden Kosten infolge der in Anspruch genommenen Gesundheitsleistungen durch den Patienten selbst.

Die weiteren Teilnehmer im Gesundheitssystem Bulgariens, die in ihrem überwiegenden Teil Nachfolger von Organisationsstrukturen geschaffen während des Aufbaus des bulgarischen Gesundheitssystem in der kommunistischen Zeit sind und nun einen neuen oder geänderten Umfang von Verantwortungen und Kompetenzen haben, sind wie folgt (für die komplette Organisationsstruktur siehe Anhang 1, Organisationsstruktur des Gesundheitssystems Bulgariens):

1. Der Ministerrat an der Staatsregierung – unter seinen Verantwortungen fällt auch die nationale Gesundheitspolitik. Auf Vorschlag des Gesundheitsministers genehmigt er die nationale Gesundheitsstrategie, die danach vom Parlament verabschiedet wird. Wieder auf Vorschlag des Gesundheitsministers genehmigt er auch die nationalen Gesundheitsprogramme. *„Die nationale Gesundheitspolitik und die nationalen Gesundheitsprogramme beruhen auf die Beurteilung des Gesundheitszustandes und der Gesundheitsbedürfnisse der Bürger, die gesundheitsdemographischen Tendenzen und die Ressourcemöglichkeiten des nationalen Gesundheitssystems"* (Art. 3 (4), das Gesetz über die Gesundheit vom 10.08.2004, in Kraft vom 01.01.2005). Die nationalen Gesundheitsprogramme werden vom Staatsbudget wie differenzierte vom Budget des Gesundheitsministeriums Ausgaben finanziert und dürfen durch alternative Finanzierungsquellen unterstützt werden (Art 3(5), das Gesetz über die Gesundheit).

2. Das Gesundheitsministerium – ihm ist das ganze Gesundheitssystem, inkl. das komplette System der Krankenhäuser und (Poly-) Kliniken unterstellt (siehe Anhang 1). Seine Verantwortung ist die Ausarbeitung der nationalen Gesundheitspolitik, das Bestimmen ihrer Ziele und Prioritäten, die Aufsicht auf das gesamte Gesundheitssystem, der Entwurf von Gesetzen. Der Gesundheitsminister leitet das nationale Gesundheitssystem und die Aufsicht auf die Tätigkeiten des Gesundheitsschutzes der Bürger (Art.5(1)1, das Gesetz über die Gesundheit), der Notfallhilfe, der transfusionalen Hämatologie, der stationären psychiatrischen Hilfe, der medizinisch-sozialen Sorge um Kinder bis zum Alter von 3 Jahren, der Transplantationen und der Gesundheitsinformation (Art.5(1)2), der Gewährleistung und der nachhaltigen Entwicklung der Gesundheitsarbeit in den Kranken- und Gesundheitseinrichtungen (Art.5(1)3) und der medizinischen Expertise (Art.5(1)4).
3. Der Höhere Medizinrat zum Gesundheitsminister – er ist ein Beratungsorgan, der aus 5 vom Gesundheitsminister ernannten Mitgliedern, 5 Vertretern des Bulgarischen Ärztlichen Verbandes, 3 Vertretern des Bulgarischen Zahnärztlichen Verbandes, 3 Vertretern der Nationalen Krankenkasse und je einem Vertreter der Nationalvereinigung der Gemeinden, der Medizinfakultäten zu den Universitäten, und des Bulgarischen Roten Kreuzes besteht (Art.6(2), das Gesetz über die Gesundheit).
4. Das Finanzministerium – es überwacht die Finanzierung des Gesundheitssektors und wirkt bei der Bestimmung der Ziele der Gesundheitspolitik und –strategie mit. Es ist ferner auch Partei in den Darlehenverträgen geschlossen mit dem Ziel der externen Finanzierung zur Unterstützung der Reformen im Gesundheitssystem (Koulaksazov et al. 2003: 14).
5. Das Wissenschafts- und Ausbildungsministerium – zu seinen Verantwortungen gehören sowohl die Ausbildungsregelungen und –inhalt, nach denen die Medizinspezialisten in den Medizinfakultäten ausgebildet werden und die Regelungen, nach denen sie ihren Beruf auf das Territorium Bulgariens ausüben dürfen (Art. 174-196) und die Medizinforschung durchgeführt wird (Art.197-209), als auch die Informationsversorgung in den Schulen und die diesbezügliche Einführung von neuen Gesundheitsausbildungsprogrammen, einschl. Vorsorge und Sport, zur Förderung eines selbstverantwortlichen Verhaltens und gesundheitskonformen Lebensstil der Bürger.
6. Das Verteidigungsministerium – unter seiner administrativen Leitung sind die Krankenhäuser und die Polykliniken für die im nationalen Verteidigungssektor beschäftigten bulgarischen Bürger.

3. Probleme und Herausforderungen vor dem bulgarischen Gesundheitssystem mit Rücksicht auf seinen bevorstehenden EU-Beitritt in 2007

3.1. Strukturänderungen. Seit dem 1991 begann ein fortlaufender Prozess der Dezentralisierung des zuvor stark zentralisierten bulgarischen Gesundheitssystem. Dieser Prozess widerspiegelte sich in drei Gruppen von Restrukturierungsmaßnahmen:

1. Der Eigentum der meisten Einrichtungen des Gesundheitssektors wurde auf die lokalen Gemeinden übertragen. Mit der Veränderung des Gesundheitsgesetzes im 1997 wurde es möglich, dass die Gesundheitseinrichtungen zu unabhängigen juristischen Personen werden und als solche fungieren.
2. Das Gesundheitsministerium baute in 1995 einen wesentlichen Teil der zentralen Administration ab und übertrug einen großen Teil der administrativen Tätigkeiten auf die 28 regionalen Gesundheitszentren.
3. Es zog einen extensiven Privatisierungsprozess der Apotheken und vieler ärztlichen Praxis. Das pharmazeutische Staatsmonopolunternehmen wurde nach einem geographischen Prinzip in 28 getrennten voneinander staatlich besitzten Unternehmen transformiert. Um Jahrhundertwende war der Eigentum auf die letzteren bis zu 70% privat.

Das Gesundheitsministerium behielt die Zentralkontrolle auf nationaler Ebene, sowie auch auf die regionalen Großkrankenhäuser (Koulaksazov et al. 2003: 23-24). Einige der schwerwiegendsten Probleme, die diese Strukturtransformationsprozesse begleitten oder aber die als Ergebnis von den letzteren entstanden sind:

- Finanzierungs- und Kontrollelücken im gesamten Gesundheitssektor, mangelnde Transparenz und unausreichende Auskunft auf dem Gesundheitsmarkt – beispielsweise in bezug auf vorwiegend aus der EU (vor allem aus Deutschland) und der Schweiz importierte Arzneimittel, welche in den späten 90er Jahren in dem sich gut ausgedehnten Netz von Privatapotheken erhältlich waren, ohne Andeutung, ob sie als rezeptpflichtig oder als rezeptfrei zu verkaufen sind. Ein weiterer Beispiel ist die neulich getroffene Entscheidung des Gesundheitsministerium, die Subventionen für alle Krankenhäuser zu kürzen, welche die im voraus geplante Anzahl von behandelten Patienten überschritten und an mehr Patienten Gesundheitsleistungen erbracht haben. Das Ziel sollte dabei sein, die Anzahl der fiktiv von den Krankenhäusern für die Ziele der Subventionssicherung angemeldeten Patienten, sowie auch die Anzahl der

Patienten, die keine bewiesene Bedürftigkeit von Krankhausbehandlung haben, begrenzt zu werden (http://www.btv.bg/news/newsprint.php?story=36977, 01.11.2004).

- ein rasantes Qualitätssinken der an Patienten erbrachten Gesundheitsleistungen in vielen kleineren Krankenhäusern, besonders in ländlicheren Orten als Folge der reduzierten Finanzierung, der Kürzungen im Gesundheitspersonal, der gesunkenen Aufsichtskontrolle und der in Bulgarien herrschenden schweren allgemeinen Wirtschaftskrise in den frühen und mittleren 90er Jahre.

- Sach- und Resourcemissbrauch seitens vieler Ärzte – der letztere entstand als Folge von der temporären gesetzlichen Lücke im Laufe der 90er Jahre, die das parallele Betreiben des ärztlichen Berufs zum einen im Rahmen eines Anstellungsverhältnisses mit Krankenhäusern und zum anderen durch die Eröffnung eigener privaten ärztlichen Praxis ermöglichte. Infolge dessen wurden kostspielige und von den noch staatlichen Krankenhäusern beschaffene Medikamente und weitere Behandlungsmaterialen in den privaten Praxis der Ärzte benutzt gegen Zahlung out-of-pocket seitens der Patienten, die Patienten wurden von den Krankenhäusern und den Polykliniken durch die behauptete Mangel an Resourcen zu den Privatpraxis und Privatkliniken umgesteuert, die teuere Medizintechnik in den Krankenhäusern wurde oft auch für die Privatpatienten der Ärzte benutzt – gegen hohe Barzahlungen des Patienten am Arzt und gegen keine Zahlung des Arztes ans Krankenhaus. Dadurch wurde der Weg der Korruption eröffnet, die mit einer absteigenden Kraft immer noch ein Problem des bulgarischen Gesundheitssystem ist. In den letzten Jahren wurden die ersten Gerichtsurteile gegen korrumpierte Ärzte, einschl. Chirurgen, gegeben, die unter anderem auch Gefängnis als Straffmaßnahme verordnen (http://www.btv.bg/news/newsprint.php?story=37127, 08.11.2004).

3.2. Finanzierung (siehe Anhang 6). Bis 2000 wurde das Gesundheitssystem aus den allgemeinen Steuern von zwei Hauptquellen finanziert – das Staats- und das Gemeindebudgets. Wie schon erwähnt, enthielt die Finanzierung des Sektors auch eine Barzahlungskomponente, die leicht in ‚under-the-table' Zahlungen überging. Nach Verabschieden des Krankenversicherungsgesetzes in 1998 (als Anhang 7 hierzu beigelegt) wurde die Finanzierung des Gesundheitssystems aufgrund Krankenversicherungsbeiträge eingeführt. Die letzteren sind zwischen Arbeitgebern und Arbeitnehmern eingeteilt. Das Niveau des Beitrags ist als Prozent vom gesetzlichen Minimalmonatsentgelt festgelegt. Ursprünglich betrug es 6% und wurde in Proportion 5:1 zulasten des Arbeitgebers eingeteilt. Momentan ist das Beitragsniveau 10%. Bis zum Beitritt Bulgariens zur

EU in 2007 soll die Beteiligung des Arbeitgebers weiter spürbar gesenkt werden und das Proportionsverhältnis 1:1 erreichen (siehe Anhang 7, Art. 40 (1)a des Krankenversicherungsgesetzes). Einige der wesentlichsten Probleme, die aus dem Übergang zu Krankenversicherungsfinanzierung entstanden sind, sind wie folgt:

- Die Selbständigen sollten alleine den gesamten Beitrag der Nationalkrankenkasse regelmäßig bezahlen. Wie auch in Deutschland der Fall ist, macht ein großer Teil von ihnen dies nicht. Es fehlen also effiziente Mechanismen zur Sicherung gegen Gesundheitsrisiko dieser Bevölkerungsgruppe, besonders in den Bedingungen einer noch stark stagnierten und im Laufe von 15 Übergangsjahren durch eine tiefe Wirtschaftskrise bedingten Volkswirtschaft. Das Problem ist besonders gravierend in bezug auf kleine Familienunternehmen, im dessen Falle kein Mitglied der Familie gegen Krankheitsrisiko versichert sein kann.
- Eine weitere Gruppe sind die Arbeitslosen, die von Krankenversicherungsbeiträgen befreit sind und die Gesundheitsleistungen zulasten des Steuerzahlers in Anspruche nehmen.
- Eine dritte Gruppe ist die zweitgrößte Minderheit Bulgariens – die Sinti und Roma[*]. Charakteristisch für diese Bevölkerungsgruppe ist die mangelnde Qualifikation, das weit verbreitete Unwillen zur Ausbildung, die daraus resultierende Besetzung der am niedrigsten bezahlten Arbeitsstellen und das hohe Risiko von Arbeitslosigkeit. Das Ergebnis ist, dass der größte Teil dieser Minderheit über Jahre lang arbeitslos ist und Sozialhilfe empfängt. Als solche bezahlen die Sinti und Roma keine Krankenversicherungsbeiträge und nutzen weiterhin, wie von den Jahrzehnten vor dem Übergang daran angewöhnt, die Gesundheitsleistungen kostenlos – nun aber schon aufgrund des Solidaritätsprinzips zulasten der anderen Beitragszahlende und des Steuerzahlers. Dies ist beachtlich besonders aus einer langfristigen Sicht, da die Geburtenraten bei den Sinti und Roma sehr hoch und der Zuwachs der Minderheit schnell ist – im Unterschied zum Rest der Bevölkerung Bulgariens, der sich durch negative Zuwachsraten kennzeichnet. Bei der bis 2007 gesetzlich festgelegten Erhöhung der vom Krankenversicherten selbst zu tragenden monatlichen Beitragszahlungen an die nationalen Krankenkasse kommt es zu leicht vorhersagbaren Finanzierungs- und Sozialvertragsproblemen im Gesundheitssektor.

---

[*] Nach offiziellen Angaben stellt sie 4,6% der Gesamtbevölkerung dar (laut Volkszählung 2001, zitiert in Bulgarien, http://de.wikipedia.org/wiki/Bulgarien, 16.01.2005), obwohl ihre Zahl viel höher (und laut mancher internationalen Quellen bis Doppel so hoch sein sollte – z.B. Büchsenschütz, 1997: 43 oder http://www.kath-zigeunerseelsorge.de, 24.10.2004) und statistisch nicht reflektierbar ist, infolge dessen, dass sich viele Angehörige dieser Minderheit entweder als Bulgaren oder als Türken je nach der Glaubensangehörigkeit bestimmen.

Laut einer Bevölkerungsuntersuchung vom Ende 2001 76% der Bevölkerung sei an der Nationalen Krankenkasse krankenversichert, 18% sei gar nicht versichert und 6% wisse es nicht, ob man krankenversichert sei oder aber nicht. Das Sinken des Anteils der durch ihre Beiträge das Gesundheitssystem finanziell unterstützenden Bürger sei auf diese drei Gruppen, vorwiegend aber auf die Minderheit der Sinti und Roma zurückzuführen (Noema, Ltd., zitiert in Koulaksazov et al. 2003: 26).

3.3. Die nationale Krankenkasse. Die Nationale Krankenkasse garantiert die Finanzierung eines Grundpakets von Gesundheitsleistungen, um dessen Umfang sie auf jährliche Basis mit den Organisationen der Medizinberufe verhandelt. In den letzten 2-3 Jahren wird ein deutlicher Trend zur andauernden Kürzungen des Grundpakets beobachtbar. Für alle Leistungen, die außerhalb des letzteren fallen, bezahlt der Patient privat und bar. Dies umreißt die Grenzen des steigenden Krankheitsrisikos, dem die Krankenversicherten ausgesetzt sind. Das Problem ist noch schärfer aus der Sicht der Tatsache, dass keine Zusatzkrankenversicherungen in Bulgarien angeboten werden. Diese Marktnische ist noch völlig unentwickelt. Eine weitere Lücke stellen die Auslandsversicherungen, die in einem sehr begrenzten Umfang zu sehr hohen für das Bulgarische Preisniveau Preisen angeboten werden. Eine vierte Problemsituation stellen die chronischen Erkrankungen, die nicht immer zu 100% ins Grundpaket der nationalen Krankenkasse aufgenommen werden. Für Patienten, die bestimmte komplizierte chirurgische Interventionen brauchen, welche aber in Bulgarien nicht durchgeführt werden, besteht in der Regel keine Sicherung durch die Krankenkasse, d.h. sie sind darauf hingewiesen, entweder privat die kompletten Kosten für Behandlung im Ausland zu tragen, oder auf Privatspenden durch die Öffentlichkeit zu hoffen. Die weiteren Restriktionen im Gesundheitsschutzniveau der bulgarischen Bürger wurden neulich vom bulgarischen Staatspräsidenten auch stark kritisiert, wobei betont wurde, das dies keine Berücksichtigung, sondern eine Verletzung des Gesetzes darstellen sollte (http://www.btv.bg/news/newsprint.php?story=37129, 08.11.2004).

Aus der Sicht des EU-Beitritts Bulgariens in 2007 stellen alle diese Problembereiche, die nicht die einzigen bestehenden Probleme im bulgarischen Gesundheitssektor sind, die Frage, inwieweit ist die Gesundheitspolitik für die bulgarischen Bürger als europäischen ‚Mehrwert' erfahrbar gemacht worden und ob sie ihnen das im Art.152 EGV vorausgesetzte hohe Gesundheitsschutzniveau sicherstellen kann. Des weiteren verdient ernste wissenschaftlich fundierte Erforschung die Frage, ob die Organisation und die Finanzierung des bulgarischen Gesundheitswesens als nationale Kompetenz EU-konform auf Dauer wären.

Benutzte Literatur:

BTV news, Ab heute reduzierte Subventionen für Krankenhäuser mit mehr Patienten, (in Bulgarischer Sprache), http://www.btv.bg/news/newsprint.php?story=36977, 01.11.2004

BTV news, Gefängnis für ein Plovdiver Chirurg angeklagt wegen Korruption (in Bulgarischer Sprache), http://www.btv.bg/news/newsprint.php?story=37127, 08.11.2004

BTV news, Der Staatspräsident Georgi Parvanov hat die Gesundheitsreform kritisiert, (in Bulgarischer Sprache), http://www.btv.bg/news/newsprint.php?story=37129, 08.11.2004

Bulgarien, in Wikipedia Enzyklopädie, http://de.wikipedia.org/wiki/Bulgarien, 16.01.2006

Bulgarische Nationale Krankenkasse, offizielle Webseite, http://www.nhif.bg/bg/default.phtml, http://www.nhif.bg/eng/default.phtml, 07.01.2005

Büchsenschütz, U. (1997), Minderheitenpolitik in Bulgarien Magisterarbeit, online Veröffentlichung vom 01.06.2004, Digitale Osteuropa-Bibliothek: Geschichte 8, ISSN 1613-1061

Das Gesetz über die Gesundheit, verabschiedet am 10.08.2004, in Kraft vom 01.01.2005, auf der Webseite der Bulgarischen Nationalen Krankenkasse, http://www.nhif.bg/bg/default.phtml, 07.01.2005

Das Krankenversicherungsgesetz vom 1998, auf der Webseite der Bulgarischen Nationalen Krankenkasse, http://www.nhif.bg/eng/default.phtml, 07.01.2005

Geschichte des Gesundheitswesens in Bulgarien (in Bulgarischer Sprache), auf der Webseite der Bulgarischen Nationalen Krankenkasse, http://www.nhif.bg/bg/default.phtml, 07.01.2005

Katholische Zigeuner Seelsorge im Auftrag der Deutschen Bischofskonferenz, Webseite, http://www.kath-zigeunerseelsorge.de, 24.10.2004

Koulaksazov, S., Todorova, S., Tragakes, E., Hristova, S. (2003), Health Care Systems in Transition, Bulgaria, European Observatory on Health Care Systems, Copenhagen, ISSN 1020-9077 Vol. 5 No. 2

Noema, Ltd., Public opinion on the health reform, December 2001, zitiert in Koulaksazov et al. 2003: 26

Anhang 1

Organisationsstruktur des Gesundheitssystems Bulgariens
(Quelle: Koulaksazov et al. 2003: 12)

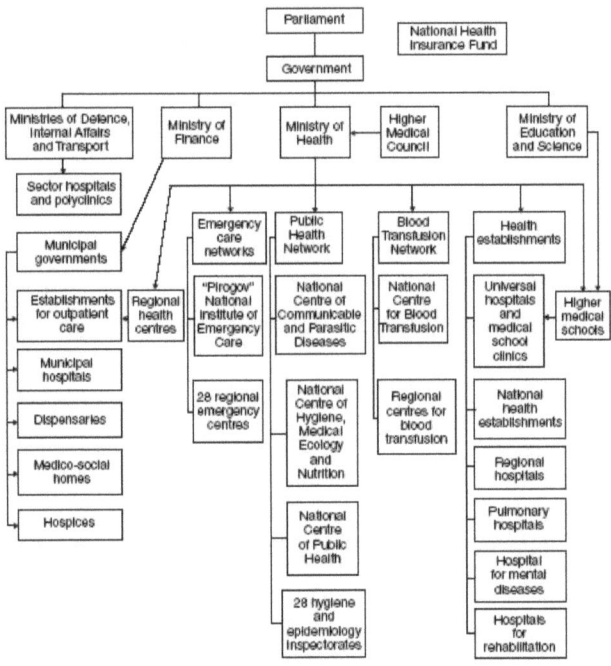

Anhang 2

Gesamtausgaben für Gesundheitsleistungen in Europa – gemessen als % vom BIP

(Quelle: Koulaksazov et al. 2003: 37)

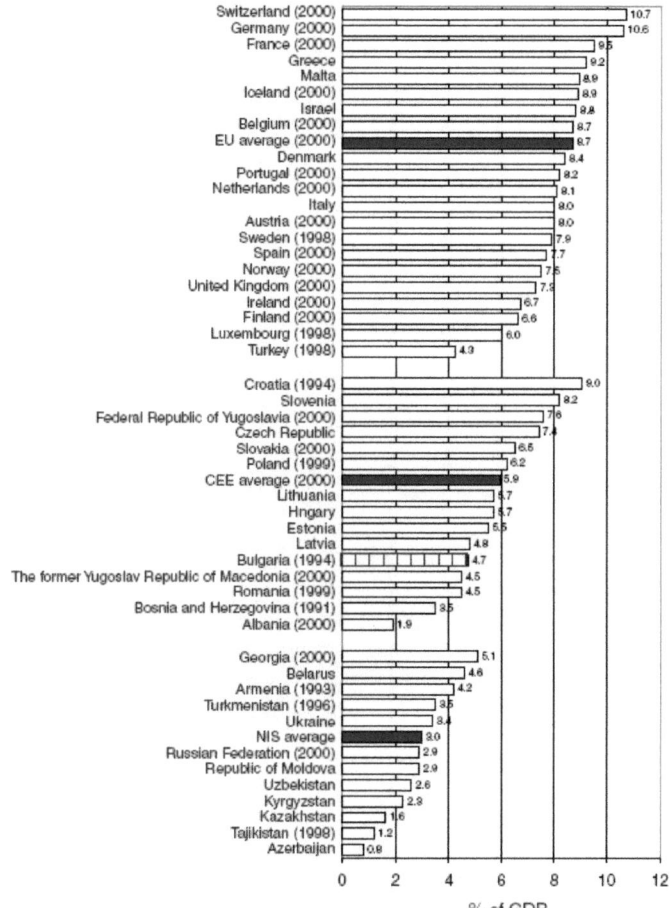

Anhang 3

Ausgaben für Gesundheitsleistungen in Europa – gemessen in USD pro Kopf

(Quelle: Koulaksazov et al. 2003: 39)

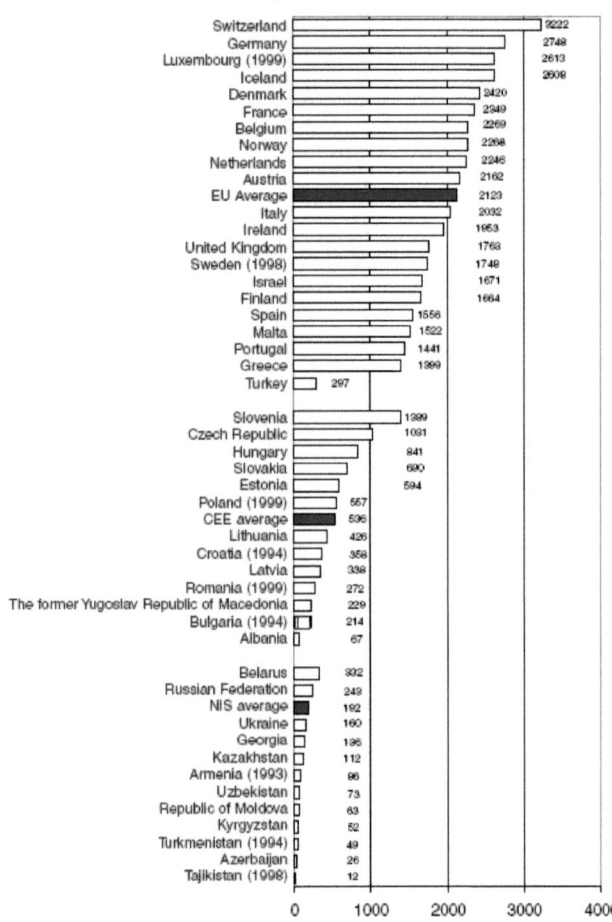

Anhang 4

Anteil der Ärzte und der Krankenschwester in Europa – gemessen pro 1000 Einwohner

(Quelle: Koulaksazov et al. 2003: 62)

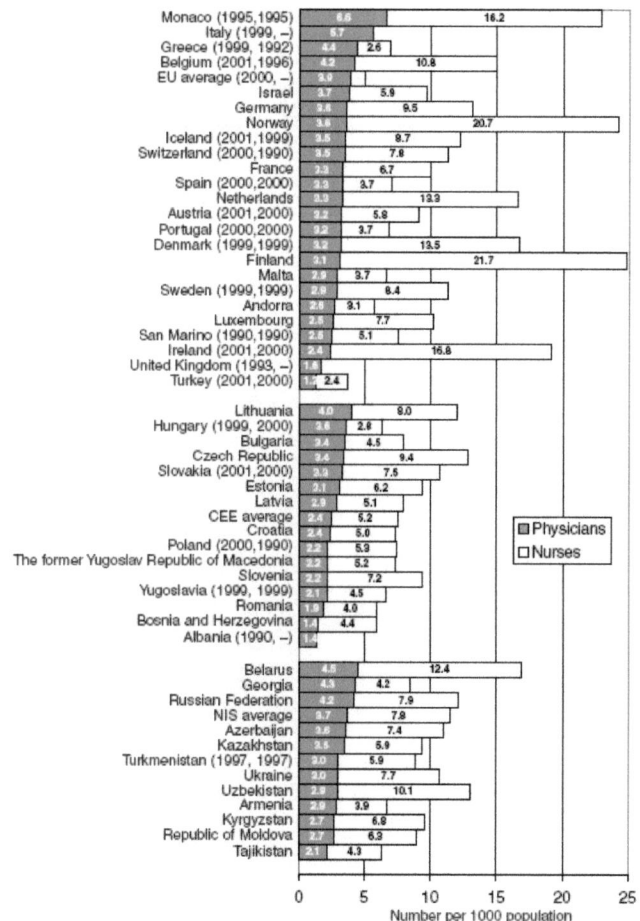

Anhang 5

Anteil des medizinischen Personals in Bulgarien – gemessen als Anteil pro 1000 Einwohner

(Quelle: Koulaksazov et al. 2003: 64)

Health care personnel, population ratio, 1980–2000

Per 1000 population	1980	1985	1990	1995	1996	1997	1998	1999	2000
Physicians	2.46	2.86	3.29	3.47	3.54	3.45	3.46	3.45	3.38
Dentists	0.54	0.64	0.70	0.65	0.66	0.63	0.59	0.57	0.83
Certified Nurses	6.85	7.40	7.67	7.68	7.72	5.71	5.75	5.52	3.86
Midwives	0.89	0.87	0.84	0.79	0.79	0.71	0.71	0.71	0.51
Pharmacists	0.41	0.47	0.49	0.22	0.22	0.19	0.19	0.19	0.13
Physicians Graduating	0.15	0.17	–	–	–	–	–	–	–
Nurses Graduating	0.55	0.13	0.16	–	–	–	–	–	–

Source: WHO Regional Office for Europe health for all database *(4)*; Ministry of Health *(14)*.

Anhang 6

Finanzierung des Gesundheitssystems Bulgariens

(Quelle: Koulaksazov et al. 2003: 68)

Financing flow chart

Anhang 7

Das Krankenversicherungsgesetz vom 1998

(Quelle: http://www.nhif.bg/eng/default.phtml, 07.01.2005)

HEALTH INSURANCE ACT

/Translation from Bulgarian/
Promulgated in State Gazette No 70 of 1998

Chapter I. GENERAL PROVISIONS
Art. 1. This law settles the health insurance in Republic of Bulgaria and the public relations connected with it.
Art. 2. The health insurance is compulsory and voluntary.
Art. 3. (1) The compulsory health insurance is a system for social health protection of the population guaranteeing a package of health services and shall be carried out by the National Health Insurance Fund (NHIF) and by its territorial divisions - Regional Health Insurance Funds (RHIF).
(2) The voluntary health insurance is additional and it shall be carried out by shareholder companies registered according to the Commercial Law and who have obtained licence under the conditions and by the order of this law.

Chapter II. COMPULSORY HEALTH INSURANCE
Section I. General Provisions
Art. 4. The compulsory health insurance guarantees to the insured persons accessible medical care and a choice of provider of such care, who has concluded contract with a Regional Health Insurance Fund.
Art. 5. The compulsory health insurance shall be carried out on the principles of:
1. compulsory participation;
2. participation of the insured persons and the employers in the management of NHIF;
3. solidarity of the insured persons in using the raised resources;
4. responsibility of the insured persons for their own health;
5. equality in using medical care;
6. self-management of NHIF;
7. contracting the relations between NHIF and the providers of the medical care;
8. publicity of the activity of NHIF.
Section II. National Health Insurance Fund
Art. 6. (1) Established is National Health Insurance Fund as a corporate body with headquarters in Sofia and subject of activity – conduct of the compulsory health insurance.
(2) The National Health Insurance Fund consists of Central Management, Regional Health Insurance Funds and their divisions in municipalities and with residences according to a list determined by the Council of Ministers.
(3) Bodies of management of NHIF are:
1. the Assembly of Representatives;
2. the Managing Board;
3. the Control Board;
4. the Director.
(4) The National Health Insurance Fund cannot carry out voluntary health insurance.
Art. 7. (1) The Assembly of Representatives shall consist of 18 representatives of each of the insured persons, the employers and the state. The quota of the insured persons shall include 6 representatives of the representative organisations acknowledged according to Art. 3 of the Labour Code.
(2) The representatives of the employers in the assembly shall be elected by the representative organisations of the employers.
(3) The representatives of the representative organisations of the workers and employees shall be elected by themselves.
(4) The representatives of the state shall be appointed by the Council of Ministers.
(5) The representatives of the insured persons shall be elected one person for each of the regions by an Assembly of Representatives of the municipalities in the respective region with the exception of Sofia city, Plovdiv and Varna regions where two representatives each shall be elected.

(6) The municipal councils shall appoint one representative for the municipality for participation in the assembly of the region, with the exception of the municipalities Plovdiv and Varna, which shall elect three representatives each.

(7) For Sofia city the municipal council shall determine one representative each for the region for participation in the assembly of Sofia city.

(8) The regional governors shall organise the assembly for carrying out the elections in the respective region.

(9) The mandate of the Assembly of Representatives shall be 4 years.

Art. 8. The Assembly of Representatives:

1. adopts, supplements and amends the Regulations for the structure and activity of the NHIF and promulgates it in the State Gazette;

2. elects and releases the members of the Managing and Control Board, determines their remuneration and adopts the regulations for their operation;

3. adopts, supplements and amends the Regulations for the structure and activity of the RHIF at the proposal of the Managing Board.

4. approves the draft law for the annual budget of NHIF;

5. approves the annual accountancy statement of NHIF;

6. releases or not from responsibility the Managing Board for the accountancy period.

Art. 9. (1) Regular meeting of the Assembly of Representatives shall be convened at least once a year by the Managing Board by a written invitation to its members. The invitation shall be promulgated in the State Gazette and in two central daily newspapers. It must indicate the date which cannot be earlier than 15 days after the promulgation, the time and the place of the meeting and the draft agenda. The materials for the draft agenda shall be sent at least 10 days before the date of holding the meeting.

(2) The assembly shall elect chairman and secretary who shall make up a list of those present and shall sign written statements for the meeting.

Art. 10. Extraordinary meeting of the Assembly of Representatives shall be convened at the request of at least one third of its members, of the Chairman of the Managing or the Control Boards or at the request of at least half plus one of the members of these boards.

Art. 11. (1) The meeting of the Assembly of Representatives shall be held if two thirds of its members are present. If there is no quorum the meeting shall be postponed by two hours and shall be held if at least one half of the members are present.

(2) The Assembly of Representatives shall take decisions by a majority of at least half plus one of those present and in the cases under Art. 8, item 1, 4 and 5 - by a majority of at least two thirds of those present.

Art. 12. (1) Release ahead of term of a member of the Assembly of Representatives shall be carried out upon filing his request, in case of death or for reasons of practical impossibility of fulfilment of his duty for a period more than one year.

(2) In the place of a released member shall be elected a new member of the Assembly by the order of Art. 7. His mandate shall end with the mandate of the Assembly of Representatives.

Art. 13. Members of the Managing Board can be elected as members of the Assembly of Representatives as well as persons who are not its members.

Art. 14. (1) The Managing Board shall be elected for a period of 4 years. The number of its members shall be nine. They shall elect among themselves chairman of the Managing Board.

(2) The Managing Board shall hold regular meetings at least once a month.

(3) Extraordinary meetings of the Managing Board can be convened by its Chairman, by one third of its members, by the Director of NHIF and by the chairman of the Control Board.

(4) The Managing Board shall work in compliance with the law, the Regulations for the structure and activity of NHIF and the Regulations for the activity of the Managing Board.

Art. 15. (1) The Managing Board:

1. together with the Director of NHIF, represents NHIF in the negotiations for working out the National Framework Contract (NFC) and signs it;

2. accepts the budget statement of NHIF and presents it to the Assembly of Representatives for approval;

3. prepares a draft law for the annual budget of NHIF and presents it to the Assembly of Representatives for approval;

4. presents at the Council of Ministers the draft law for the annual budget of NHIF;

5. holds a competition, according to the Labour Code, for a Director of NHIF, upon which the Chairman of the Managing Board concludes employment contract with the winner of the competition;

6. takes decisions for concluding rental contracts;

7. promulgates in the State Gazette the NFC.

(2) The Managing Board shall take decisions in the presence of at least two thirds of its members, but by no less than 5 "pro" votes.

(3) The members of the Managing Board shall be jointly responsible for damages caused to NHIF through their fault.

(4) The director of NHIF shall participate in the meetings of the Managing Board.
Art. 16. As members of the Control Board shall be elected only members of the Assembly of Representatives.
Art. 17. (1) The Control Board shall be elected for a period of 4 years. The number of its members shall be five. They shall elect among themselves the Chairman of the Board.
(2) The control body shall exercise general control over the activity of the Managing Board, the Director of NHIF and the Directors of RHIF.
(3) The Control Board shall work in compliance with the acting legislation and the Regulations of NHIF.
(4) The Control Board shall meet at least once in 3 months and shall be convened by the Chairman or at the request of two of its members. Its decisions shall be taken if a quorum of four of its members is available, by an open voting and a majority of at least half plus one of the present members. Non-participation in the voting shall not be admitted.
(5) The members of the Control Board cannot be elected for mo re than two mandates.
Art. 18. (1) Members of the Assembly of Representatives, of the Managing Board and the Control Board cannot be persons who are:
1. members of the Parliament or ministers;
2. medical care executives under this law;
3. members of managing or control bodies of other organisations carrying out insurance activity;
4. directors of RHIF, their spouses or relatives on descending and collateral line up to fourth degree including;
5. persons having been members of managing or control bodies of trade company or unlimited responsible partners in companies which are closed due to insolvency whereupon unsatisfied creditors have remained;
6. sole entrepreneurs who have got into insolvency whereupon unsatisfied creditors have remained;
7. persons deprived of the right to occupy materially responsible positions;
8. persons having been convicted for premeditated crime of general nature.
(2) One person cannot be simultaneously member of the Managing and Control Boards;
Art. 19. The Director of NHIF:
1. represents NHIF within the frames of the authorities given to him by the Managing Board;
2. organises and manages the activity of NHIF in compliance with the law, the Regulations for the structure and activity of NHIF, the decisions of the Assembly of Representatives and of the Managing Board;
3. concludes, amends and discontinues the contracts with the directors of RHIF and with the employees of the Central Management of NHIF;
4. works out the draft law for the annual budget of NHIF and the report on the activity and presents them to the Managing Board.
Art. 20. The Director of RHIF:
1. represents NHIF on territorial level within the frames of the authorities given to him by the Managing Board of NHIF;
2. organises and manages the activity of RHIF in compliance with the law, the Regulations for the structure and activity of NHIF, the decisions of the Assembly of Representatives, of the Managing Board, of the Director of NHIF and the Regulations for the structure and activity of RHIF;
3. concludes, amends and discontinues the contracts with the employees of the respective RHIF;
4. concludes, amends and discontinues the contracts with the medical care executives on the territory serviced by RHIF according to the law, the NFC and the Regulations for the structure and activity of NHIF and RHIF respectively.
Art. 21. The Director of NHIF and the directors of RHIF, as well as the persons under Art. 18 cannot be members of the managing bodies of trade companies, co-operations and non-profit associations providing medical care.
Section III. Financial structure of the National Health Insurance Fund
Art. 22. The budget of NHIF is a basic financial plan for raising and spending of the monetary resources of the compulsory health insurance and is separagraphted from the state budget.
Art. 23. (1) The revenue of NHIF are raised from:
1. insurance contributions;
2. interest and receipts from the management of the property of the Fund;
3. revenues stipulated by other laws in favour of the health insurance;
4. reimbursement of insurance expenses in the cases stipulated by normative acts;
5. fines and penalty interest;
6. taxes determined by a tariff of the Council of Ministers;
7. liquidation shares of trade companies - debtors, declared for liquidation;
8. donations and inheritance;
9. other sources.
(2) In cases of shortage of resources, short-term interest free loans from the republican budget or credits from other institutions can be used.
Art. 24. The resources of NHIF shall be spent for:

1. payment of medical care according to Art. 45, contracted by the NFC and by the contracts with the executives;
2. support of the administrative activities related to the health insurance stipulated by the annual budget law of NHIF;
3. publishing activity within the frames of the resources for support of the administrative activities of NHIF;
4. acquisition of movable property and real estates and other investment expenditures for the needs of NHIF;
5. other expenses.

Art. 25. The National Health Insurance Fund shall form an compulsory reserve.

Art. 26. (1) The reserve of NHIF shall be raised from:
1. five percent of the collected insurance contributions;
2. other revenue.

(2) The resources of the reserve shall be used for expenses in case of a considerable deviations from the even spending of the resources or of territorial misbalance of the use of medical care.

(3) The total amount of the reserve cannot exceed 15 percent of the annual revenue of NHIF calculated as average arithmetic value of the annual revenue for the preceding 3 years.

Art. 27. (1) The budget of NHIF shall be worked out and realised in a such way that the expenses shall not exceed the revenue within the frames of one budget year.

(2) The temporary free resources and the resources of the reserve of NHIF can be deposited in bank accounts and in state securities.

(3) The banks having the right to operate with the resources of NHIF shall be determined jointly by the Bulgarian National Bank and the Ministry of Finance. Among the banks determined by the Bulgarian National Bank and the Ministry of Finance the Managing Board of NHIF shall choose those to which it shall assign the right to operate with the resources of NHIF.

Art. 28. First degree administrator with the resources of NHIF shall be the Director of NHIF and the directors of RHIF shall be second degree administrators with them.

Art. 29. (1) The Managing Board of NHIF shall present at the Council of Ministers a draft law for the budget of NHIF within the period stipulated for presentation of a draft law for the state budget of the Republic of Bulgaria for the next calendar year.

(2) The draft law for the annual budget of NHIF shall be considered by the National Assembly simultaneously with the draft laws for the state budget and for the budget of the state public insurance.

(3) The law for the budget of NHIF shall determine the rate of the health insurance contribution.

(4) In case that the draft law of the budget of the National Health Insurance Fund is not adopted by the National Assembly until the beginning of the budget year, the insurance income shall be collected and the insurance expenses shall be made according to the budget approved for the preceding year, and the spent for the support of the National Health Insurance Fund shall be monthly 1/12 of the expenses provided by the budget for the preceding year.

Art. 30. (1) The annual report on the fulfilment of the budget of NHIF shall be presented by the Managing Board through the Council of Ministers at the National Assembly for adopting together with the report on the fulfilment of the state budget.

(2) The decision of the National Assembly for adopting the report on the fulfilment of the budget of NHIF shall be promulgated in the State Gazette.

Art. 31. The National Health Insurance Fund cannot possess medical surgeries, laboratories, health establishments and pharmacies.

Art. 32. (Revoked, State Gazette, No 153 of 1998)

Section IV. Insured persons. Rights and obligations

Art. 33. Compulsory insured by the National Health Insurance Fund shall be:
1. all Bulgarian citizens who are not citizens of another country;
2. Bulgarian citizens who are also citizens of other country and permanently reside on the territory of the Republic of Bulgaria;
3. foreign citizens or persons without citizenship with permitted long-term stay on the territory of the Republic of Bulgaria, unless provided otherwise by an international agreement party to which is the Republic of Bulgaria;
4. persons with a refugee status or granted right to asylum.

Art. 34. (1) The obligation for insurance occurs:
1. for all Bulgarian citizens - from the enactment of the law and for the newly born - from the date of birth;
2. according to Art. 33, item 2 - from the date of obtaining permit for permanent residence;
3. according to Art. 33, item 3 - from the date of opening procedures for granting status of refugee or right of asylum.

(2) The rights of the insured under Art. 33 shall occur:
1. for the newly born - from the date of birth;
2. for all the others - from the date of payment of the health insurance contribution.

(3) The rights of the insured are personal and cannot be ceded (transferred).

Art. 35. The compulsory insured persons have the right:

1. to medical care within the range under Art. 45, in NFC and in the contracts between RHIF and the medical care executives;
2. to choose one medical care executive who has concluded contract with RHIF;
3. to emergency medical care wherever it is needed;
4. to receive information from RHIF about the contracts concluded by it with the medical care executives;
5. to participate in the management of NHIF through their representatives;
6. to file complaints to the director of the respective RHIF for violations of the law and the contracts.

Art. 36. (1) The compulsory insured persons have the right to receive partially or in full the value of the expenses for medical care abroad only if they have received a preliminary permit by NHIF.
(2) Permit under paragraphgraph 1 shall only be given for the types of medical care which is not provided in the country, by the order of Art. 78 and 79.

Art. 37. (1) The persons under Art. 33 shall pay to the physician, the dentist or to the health establishment sums as follows:
1. for every visit to the physician or dentist - 1 percent of the minimal salary established for the country;
2. for every day of hospital treatment - 2 percent of the minimal salary established for the country, but for no more than 20 days yearly.
(2) Exempt from payment of the sums under paragraphgraph 1 shall be persons with diseases determined according to a list to NFC, as well as minors and underage and unemployed members of the family; recruitment military men; victims as a result of or on occasion of the defence of the country, war veterans, military disabled; detained or convicted; socially week receiving help according to the Regulations for social support; persons without income accommodated in the homes for children and young persons, in homes for children of pre-school age and in the homes for social welfare.
(3) The physician, the dentist or the health establishment shall issue to the persons under paragraphgraph 1 a receipt for the paid sums.

Art. 38. The insured persons are obliged to observe the prescriptions of the medical care executives and the requirements for prophylactics of the diseases in compliance with NFC and the contracts with the executives.

Art. 39. (1) All persons who, according to this law, are obliged to pay insurance contributions shall be obliged, from the moment of occurrence of the grounds for health insurance, to present monthly data for the insured persons at the territorial divisions of the National Insurance Institute by declarations in a form approved by the National Insurance Institute and the National Health Insurance Fund.
(2) The persons insuring members of their families according to this law shall present data for them in declarations according to a form approved by the National Insurance Institute and the National Health Insurance Fund.
(3) In the cases when the persons pay contributions in advance according to this law they shall fill out declaration for the period of advance payment in a form approved by the National Insurance Institute and the National Health Insurance Fund.
(4) The foreigners who stay on short-term basis in the Republic of Bulgaria, as well as persons with dual Bulgarian and foreign citizenship who are not insured by the order of this law shall pay the value of the rendered medical care, unless an international agreement party to which is the Republic of Bulgaria is not in force for them.

Section V. Health insurance contributions

Art. 40. (1) The health insurance contribution of the insured person, determined by the order of Art. 29, paragraph 3 shall be calculated over an income and shall be paid as follows:
1. for a person receiving income from legal terms of employment or official legal terms of employment or terms of employment occurred on the basis of special laws - the taxable income under the Law for taxation of the income of individuals:
a) the contribution for the persons working under legal terms of employment shall be paid in by the employer or the administrative body and by the insured person in correlation:
 - 2000 - 2001 - 80:20;
 - 2002 - 75:25;
 - 2003 - 70:30;
 - 2004 - 65:35;
 - 2005 - 60:40;
 - 2006 - 55:45;
 - 2007 and the following years - 50:50;
b) the contribution for the persons working under official legal terms of employment and under legal terms of employment occurring on the grounds of special laws shall be paid in by the employer and shall be for the account of the state budget;
c) the employer or the administrative body shall pay in the contributions simultaneously with the payment of the remuneration; in paying the remuneration the employer or the administrative body shall deduct the contributions due by the insured persons, including the contributions for the members of the family whom they insure;

2. the sole entrepreneurs, the individuals who have established limited liability companies, the partners in trade companies, and the persons registered as freelance practitioners or craft industry shall be insured on a declared monthly income which cannot be less than the double amount of the minimal salary established in the country, and annually - on the taxable income according to the data of the tax declaration:
a) the contributions shall be paid in by the 10th of the month following the month which they concern;
b) the monthly insurance income, in view of the calculation of the annual amount of the contribution, shall be obtained as the annual taxable income is divided by the period during which the activity has been practised;
c) for annual taxation the contributions shall be paid in by the deadline for payment of the taxes under the Law for taxation of the income of individuals;
3. for the persons who do not declare income under item 2 and work without legal terms of employment under contract with assignor - enterprise or another organisation, the insurance contributions shall be paid in every month on the taxable income by the enterprise or the organisation, deducting from the paid remuneration of the person; the contributions shall be paid in by the enterprise or the organisation by the 10th of the month following the month which they concern; for these persons an annual equalisation of the income shall be made, on which the contributions under item 2, letter b and c are due;
4. for the retired - the amount of the pension or the sum of pensions, without the additions to them; the contributions shall be for the account of the state budget and shall be paid in by the 10th of the month following the month which they concern;
5. for the retired who receive pensions under international agreements, entirely for the account of a foreign insurance institute - the double amount of the minimal salary established in the country; the contributions shall be for the account of the person and shall be paid in by the 10th of the month following the month which they concern;
6. for persons receiving compensations for temporary labour incapacity due to illness, pregnancy, childbirth or raising child - the size of the compensation; the contributions shall be for the account of the employer or the administrative body and shall be equal to the part of the contribution due by him installed in payment of the compensations; when the person is insured for his account the contributions shall be paid in by the 10th of the month following the month which they concern;
7. for the persons receiving income on various grounds, indicated under item 1, 2, 3, 4, 5 and 6 the contributions shall be made on the sum of the insurance income;
8. for the persons receiving compensation for unemployment - the size of the paid compensation; the contributions shall be for the account of fund "Professional qualification and unemployment" and shall be paid in by the 10th of the month following the month which they concern;
9. for the persons and members of families with a right of social welfare and for underage persons without parents, who are not subject to insurance on other grounds - the one-time amount of the minimal salary established for the country; the contributions shall be for the account of the municipal budgets and shall be paid in by the 10th of the month following the month which they concern;
10. for parent (adopting parent) or spouse who take care for disabled with lost labour capacity over 90 percent, who permanently need help, who are not subject to insurance on other grounds - the one-time amount of the minimal salary established for the country. The contributions shall be for the account of the municipal budgets and shall be paid by the 10th of the month following the one that they regard;
11. for the conscript military servicemen; for the war veterans and for the military disabled; for disabled during or on occasion of the defence of the country, during natural calamities and accidents and for the affected in fulfilment of their official duty employees of the Ministry of Internal Affairs who are not subject to insurance on other grounds; for persons under proceedings for granting refugee status or a right of asylum; for detained or imprisoned; for persons without income, accommodated in homes for children and youth, homes for children in pre-school age and in the homes for social care; for persons studying in high schools, without income, until the accomplishment of 26 years - the one-time amount of the minimal salary established in the country; the contributions shall be paid in by the 10th of the month following the month which they concern and shall be for the account of the state budget, and shall be made by transfer through the respective administrative body or the municipal budgets;
12. for the persons using unpaid leave, who are not subject to insurance on other grounds - the one-time amount of the minimal salary established in the country; the contributions shall be for the account of the employer and shall be paid in with the payment of the remuneration by the respective enterprise or other organisation;
13. for the employees of the Bulgarian Orthodox Church and other religions acknowledged by a normative order, who have no legal terms of employment - the one-time amount of the minimal salary established in the country; the contributions shall be paid in by the 10th of the month following the month which they concern by the central management of the respective religious institution;
14. for the members of the family who are not insured - 5 percent of the contribution for every insured member of the family; the contributions shall be for the account of the insured person; when the insured person receives income under item 1, 3 and 6 the contribution shall be deducted by the employer (the enterprise, the administrative body or the

organisation with the payment of the remuneration; for the persons working under employment, official legal terms or legal terms occurring on the grounds of special laws the contributions shall be deducted and made by the employer or the administrative body with the payment of the remuneration or the pecuniary compensations; if the person is insured for his account, as well as for the persons insured according to item 3 the contributions shall be paid in by the 10th of the month following the one which they concern;

15. the persons who are not subject to insurance under item 1 - 13 shall be insured on a declared insurance income not less than the double amount of the minimal salary established in the country; the contributions shall be for their account and shall be paid in by the 10th of the month following the month which they concern; if these persons are subject to annual taxation, an annual equalisation of the contributions shall be paid in by the order of item 2.

(2) The maximal amount of the monthly income on which the health insurance contribution is due shall be 10 minimal salaries established for the country.

(3) For the persons under paragraph 1, item 7 the contributions shall be made on the sum of the insurance income by the order stipulated for the respective type of income, but totally on not more than the 10-fold amount of the minimal salary established in the country.

Art. 41. (1) The insurance contributions under this law shall be paid in to the accounts for collecting health insurance contributions in the territorial divisions of the National Insurance Institute from where they shall obligatorily be daily transferred to the raising account for health insurance contributions of the Central Management of the National Insurance Institute.

(2) The sums of health insurance contributions collected in the National Insurance Institute shall be transferred to the raising account of the National Health Insurance Fund (NHIF) by the end of every work day.

Art. 42. (1) The insurance income on which the contribution is calculated shall be established by the payrolls and other documents for paid remuneration, by the pension cards, the paid patient charts, the paid compensations for unemployed and by the tax declarations according to the Law for taxation of the income of individuals.

(2) The health insurance contribution s hall not be subject to taxation.

(3) The persons shall file declarations with the payer of the income or with the respective bodies for the members of their families whom they are obliged to insure. The annual declaration under the Law for taxation of the income of individuals shall contain the health insurance contributions paid during the year and the due sums after the annual equalisation, if any.

(4) The employers, the tax offices, the municipal authorities, the administrative bodies, the assignors and the self-insured shall be obliged to present to the National Insurance Institute and to NHIF the necessary information under Art. 42, paragraphs 1 and 3.

Art. 43. The insured persons under Art. 40, paragraph 1, item 2, 5 and 14 can pay the health insurance contributions for themselves and for the members of their family in advance, for a period chosen by them.

Art. 44. The contributions shall be paid:
1. through a bank;
2. by post order.

Section VI. Range of the medical care for the compulsory health insurance

Art. 45. (1) The National Health Insurance Fund shall pay for the following medical services:
1. medical and dental services for prevention against diseases;
2. medical and dental services for early discovery of diseases;
3. out-patient and hospital medical care for diagnostics and treatment of a disease;
4. medical rehabilitation;
5. emergency medical care;
6. medical care for pregnancy, labour and motherhood;
7. abortions for medical indications and for pregnancy as a result of rape;
8. dental services;
9. medical care in cases of home treatment;
10. medical supplies and consumption materials for home treatment;
11. medical expertise of the labour capacity;
12. transport services for medical indications;

(2) The minimal package of medical care under paragraph 1 shall be determined by the Minister of Health.

Art. 46. (1) The order providing and the extent of the medical care for the individual types of medical care under Art. 45 shall be determined by the NFC and by the contracts between RHIF and the executives.

(2) The quality of the rendered medical services, paid by NHIF must correspond to the rules for the good medical practice, which shall be adopted by the professional organisations of physicians and dentists and by NHIF and shall be approved by the Minister of Health.

(3) The rules for the good medical practice shall contain the requirements for due time, enough care and quality of the medical care.

Art. 47. The payment for the medical care rendered to the insured person shall be made by RHIF to the executive who has rendered it.

Art. 48. The NHIF shall be obliged to inform systematically the insured persons regarding the measures of protecting and improvement of their health.

Art. 49. For established labour conditions and other harmful factors of the environment which threaten the health of the insured persons the physicians - controllers shall inform immediately the employers, the bodies of labour safety, the state sanitary control, the state veterinary control and the bodies of protection of the environment for the purpose of taking the necessary measures.

Art. 50. For using medical care the insured persons shall be obliged to present their health insurance book or a document certifying the paid contributions.

Art. 51. The medical care, outside the range of Art. 45 and the contracted conditions in the NFC shall not be paid by NHIF.

Art. 52. The persons not insured under this law shall pay the medical care.

Section VII. National Framework Contract

Art. 53. For carrying out the activities under this law a National Framework Contract (NFC) shall be signed.

Art. 54. (1) The working out and signing the NFC shall be carried out by 10 representatives of NHIF and 10 representatives of the professional organisations of the physicians and dentists. The status of the professional organisations of the physicians and dentists and the order of appointment of their representatives for participation in the working out and signing of NFC shall be settled by a separate law.

(2) Representatives of NHIF for signing the NFC shall be the members of the Managing Board and the Director of the Central Management.

(3) The NFC shall be considered concluded when signed by no less than 8 representatives of NHIF and 8 representatives of the professional organisations of the physicians and dentists. The Minister of Health shall countersign the National Framework Contract.

Art. 55. (1) The representatives of NHIF and of the professional organisations of the physicians and dentists shall work out every year a NFC for the next year.

(2) The National Framework Contract shall contain:

1. the conditions and the order of determining the medical care executives with whom RHIF shall conclude contracts;
2. the individual types of medical care under Art. 45;
3. the conditions and order of rendering the service under item 2;
4. the range, the prices and the methodology of payment of the services under item 2;
5. the quality and the accessibility of the contracted medical aid;
6. the documentation and the documents circulation;
7. the lists of the medical supplies for which NHIF, partially or in full, pays contracted with the producers, distributors of medical supplies and pharmacies.
8. the obligations of the parties to the informational services and the informational exchange;
9. the conditions and the order of control over the fulfilment of the contracts;
10. other issues of importance for the health insurance;
11. sanctions for failure to fulfil the contract.

(3) If a consent is not reached in contracting the NFC within the period under paragraph 1 or in case of undue adoption of the Law for the budget of NHIF the Contract from the preceding year shall continue its effect from January 1 of the next year. In this case the prices under paragraph 2, item 4 shall be indexed by the official inflation index for the preceding year, upon which they shall be promulgated in the State Gazette. The Contract shall continue its effect until the signing of a new Contract.

(4) Upon request of whichever of the parties participating in the agreement NFC can be amended by the order of Art. 54, paragraph 1 but not more than once in 6 months.

(5) The NFC shall be promulgated in the State Gazette and shall be compulsory for NHIF and RHIF and for the executives.

(6) The inclusion in NFC of new methods of diagnostics and treatment shall be admitted by the order of Art. 31, paragraph 3 of the Law for the national health.

(7) In case that a consent is not reached in contracting the first NFC the financing of the health care shall be continued by the state budget.

Art. 56. In the contracts with NHIF the medical care executives shall undertake the responsibility to prescribe medicines from the lists under Art. 55, paragraph 2, item 7 to the insured persons.

Art. 57. When it is necessary to prescribe medical supply other than those of the lists under Art. 55, paragraph 2, item 7, the medical care executive shall inform RHIF and shall substantiate the need of this medicine. In these cases the RHIF can pay these medicines.

Section VIII. Contract between the National Health Insurance Fund and medical care executive

Art. 58. Providers of medical care in the context of this law are medical establishments according to the Law for the medical establishments and health establishments according to the Law for the national health.

Art. 59. (1) The contracts under Art. 20, item 4 for medical care under this law and in compliance with the NFC shall be concluded between the director of RHIF and the medical care executives.

(2) The contracts under paragraph 1 cannot be concluded under conditions less favourable than those adopted by NFC.

(3) The contracts under paragraph 1 shall be concluded in writing for the period of effect of the NFC and shall remain in force until the adoption of a new one or the change of the acting NFC.

(4) The contracts under paragraph 1 shall specify the requirements and the conditions stipulated by Art. 55, paragraph 2, items 2 - 11, for implementation on the respective territory. The contracts shall specify the relations between the medical care executives and between them and other persons, for fulfilment of the contracted medical care.

(5) The refusal of the director of RHIF to conclude contract with the executive can be appealed by the executive within 2 weeks before the Managing Board of NHIF through the director of NHIF if the latter does not revoke unilaterally the refusal.

(6) The Managing Board shall take decision on the refusal within 1 month from filing the appeal. The refusal shall be subject to appeal under the Law for the administrative proceedings before the respective district court within 2 months.

Art. 60. Subject to agreement and payment on the part of NHIF shall not be the scientific activity and the education of medical specialists, carried out in health establishments.

Art. 61. The director of RHIF can also conclude contracts with physicians and dentists practising out of hospitals who have contracts with a hospital on the same territory. The contract shall determine the conditions and the order of paying the medical care provided in the hospital.

Art. 62. The director of RHIF can conclude contract for out-patient treatment with physicians and dentists working in a hospital on condition that there are not enough physicians of the same speciality on the territory who are practising out of the hospitals, and the activity of the hospital is not disrupted.

Section IX. Informational provision of the activity of the National Health Insurance Fund

Art. 63. The National Health Insurance Fund shall establish an information system which shall contain:

1. a register of the insured persons including: passport data; unique identification number; grounds for insurance under Art. 33; paid contributions;

2. a register of the medical care executives with the passport and professional data of the executive, the contract concluded with him.

3. a register of producers, importers and distributors of medical supplies and pharmacies having concluded contracts with the NHIF;

4. information from the activity of the control bodies;

5. administrative information providing the activity of NHIF.

Art. 64. Every insured person shall have the right to receive from NHIF the available information about the medical care and its price received by him during the last 5 years and its price by an order determined by the fund.

Art. 65. The medical care executives shall be obliged to present to RHIF information about the activity carried out by them according to methodologies and range adopted by NFC.

Art. 66. The informational system of the compulsory health insurance shall use the codes and nomenclature for registration and accounting the health care services used in the country.

Art. 67. The data for the insured persons shall be kept in NHIF for a period of 10 years from conclusion of their health insurance, and those for the executives - 10 years from expiration of their last contract with NHIF.

Art. 68. (1) Data related to the personality of the insured can only be used for:

1. establishing the insurance relations with NHIF;

2. payment to the medical care executive;

3. issuance of health insurance book, medical or financial document;

4. establishment of sums subject to collection or reimbursement to the payer of the instalments or to the medical care executive;

5. establishment of caused damages to the insured during medical operations;

6. exercising financial control.

(2) Data related to the medical care executive can only be used for:

1. keeping register of the medical care executives;

2. payment of the medical services rendered by him;

3. exercising professional and financial control.

(3) Besides the cases under paragraph 1 and 2 NHIF can submit data to state bodies about the personality of the insured or about the executive if this is stipulated by a law.

(4) The employees of the central management of NHIF or RHIF shall not have the right to spread information related to the personality of the insured, the medical care executive or an employee except in the cases stipulated by a law.

Art. 69. The National Insurance Institute shall be obliged to provide information to the National Institute of Statistics about the insured persons and the paid health insurance contributions.

Section X. Control, expertise and disputes

Art. 70. The control over the fulfilment of the budget of NHIF shall be carried out by the Audit Office.

Art. 71. The control over the activity of the Managing Board, the Director of NHIF and the directors of RHIF shall be carried out by the Control Board according to the provisions of this law and the Regulations for the structure and activity of NHIF.

Art. 72. (1) The Director of NHIF shall carry out complete control over the activity of the health insurance.

(2) The immediate control shall be carried out by officials of RHIF - financial inspectors and physicians - controllers.

Art. 73. (1) The financial inspectors shall have the right:

1. (revoked, State Gazette No. 110/ 1999);
2. to inspect the reporting documents of the medical care executives;
3. to carry out control over the expediency of the expenditures;
4. to carry out inspections on claims of insured persons and employers.

(2) For fulfilment of the activities under paragraph 1 the financial inspectors shall have the right of access to information from the employers, the insured and the executives.

(3) The financial inspectors shall not have the right disseminate information having become known to them in connection with the activity under paragraph 1 except in the cases provided by a law.

Art. 73a. The financial control over the revenue of NHIF from health insurance contributions and the due interest shall be exercised by the control bodies of the National Insurance Institute by the order of the Code for the compulsory public insurance.

Art. 74. (1) The control related to rendering medical care should be carried out by physicians-controllers who shall have the right to inspect:

1. the compliance with the rules for good medical practice;
2. the type and the volume of the rendered medical care;
3. the type and the quantity of the prescribed medical supplies;
4. the correspondence between the rendered medical care and the paid money.

(2) The physicians-controllers shall carry out their activities on filed complaints through sudden inspections on the chance principle of 2 percent of the medical care executives within the range of every RHIF and in cases of establishing excess of the expenses for medical care by 25 percent or more for one period of six months.

(3) When establishing violations under paragraph 1, item 1 - 4 the physician-controller shall issue written statement which shall describe the established facts. The written statement shall be signed by the physician-controller. Copy of the written statement shall be submitted to the inspected person and copies of it shall be sent to the director of the respective RHIF and to the respective regional college of the professional organisation of the physicians or of the dentists.

(4) The person, subject to inspection, shall have the right to present written statement to the director of RHIF on the findings of the physician-controller within 7 days from presentation of the written statement under paragraph 3.

Art. 75. (1) In the cases when the person disputes the findings of the physician-controller the director of RHIF shall, within 7 days from receipt of the written statement under Art. 74, paragraph 4, send the dispute for settlement by an Arbitration Commission.

(2) The Arbitration Commission shall consist of 6 members - equal number of representatives of RHIF and of the regional college of the respective professional organisation of the physicians or of the dentists.

(3) The Arbitration Commission shall take decision within 1 month from receipt of the file.

Art. 76. (1) If the Arbitration Commission confirms the findings of the physician-controller shall apply the sanctions stipulated by the contract between RHIF and the medical care executive.

(2) The sanctions shall be subject to court appeal by the order of the Law for the administrative proceedings.

Art. 77. The individuals and the corporate bodies shall be obliged to submit to the control bodies of NHIF and of the National Insurance Institute the requested documents, information, references, declarations, explanations and other carriers of information related to the health insurance and to render assistance in fulfilment of their official duties.

Art. 78. The National Health Insurance Fund can perform expertise in case of necessity of:

1. medical care, if its cost exceeds 200 times the minimal monthly salary established in the country;
2. expensive medical supplies in the cases not stipulated by NFC;
3. treatment abroad.

Art. 79. The expertise under Art. 78 shall be performed by an order determined by the Regulations for the structure and activity of NHIF, by a commission in the Central Management.

Art. 80. The disputes on the fulfilment of the contracts between NHIF, RHIF and the medical care executives shall be settled by court order if agreement cannot be reached through arbitration.

Chapter III. VOLUNTARY HEALTH INSURANCE

Section I. General provisions

Art. 81. The voluntary health insurance provides for the insured persons medical and other services according to the NFC as well as beyond the range of the compulsory health insurance.

Art. 82. (1) For carrying out voluntary health insurance contracts shall be concluded between the insured and the insurance company.

(2) The contract shall contain the type and the volume of the medical and other services which are guaranteed by the assuring company to the insured, as well as the amount of the insurance premium under this contract.

(3) The employers can conclude, on their behalf and for their account, contracts for voluntary insurance for their employees and workers.

Art. 83. The prices of the medical and other services - subject to voluntary health insurance as well as the conditions and the order of their providing, shall be contracted between the assuring company and the medical care executives.

Art. 84. The contracts between the companies for voluntary health insurance and the insured persons, as well as the contracts between the companies for voluntary health insurance and the medical care executives shall be concluded in compliance with the Law for the obligations and contracts.

Art. 85. (1) Joint-stock companies can carry out voluntary health insurance only if they have received licence under the conditions and by the order of this law.

(2) Joint-stock companies can obtain licence if they are registered with subject of activity only for voluntary health insurance.

Art. 86. Joint-stock companies having obtained licence can hold medical surgeries, health establishments and pharmacies.

Art. 87. (1) Joint-stock companies for voluntary health insurance shall be established, shall carry out activities and shall be closed down by the order of the Commercial Law inasmuch as this law does not provide otherwise.

(2) The minimal amount of the capital of the joint-stock company for voluntary health insurance is 2 000 000 levs.

(3) By the moment of filing for licensing for voluntary health insurance the monetary capital must be deposited in full at the Bulgarian National Bank.

(4) When withdrawing the deposit for registration it can be replaced by apportion instalment.

Art. 88. The stock of the joint-stock companies with subject of activity voluntary health insurance can only be personal.

Art. 89. (1) Member of a Managing Board, of a Supervisory Board, of a Board of Directors can be a person meeting the requirements of the Commercial Law.

(2) Executive Director can be a person who meets the requirements of the Commercial Law as well as:

1. to have residence in the country;
2. to have higher education;
3. to have professional experience in one of the following specialities: health care, economics, law.

Art. 90. The statutes of the joint-stock company shall also state the types of health insurance to be provided by the voluntary health insurance.

Section II. Licensing for voluntary health insurance

Art. 91. Licence for voluntary health insurance shall be issued by the State Agency for Insurance Supervision.

Art. 92. (1) The types of health insurance under the voluntary health insurance are separated in the following packages of activities for:

1. health improvement and prevention of diseases;
2. out-patient medical care;
3. hospital medical care;
4. services related to communal and other additional conditions of rendering medical care;
5. reimbursement of expenses;

(2) Individual licence shall be issued for each package of activities under paragraph 1.

(3) The licence fee for one package amounts to 1 000 levs.

(4) The fee under paragraph 3 shall be paid to an account of the Ministry of Health.

Art. 93. Application for issuing licence shall be filed accompanied by:

1. decision for court registration;
2. copy of the statutes;
3. list of the stock holders;
4. programme and prognoses for the activity of the company for the first 2 years which shall contain: revenue from the insurance premiums; expenses related to servicing the insurance contracts, expenses related to the activity and the amount of the resources in fund "Reserve";
5. investment programme of the company;
6. list of the packages of activities under Art. 92, paragraph 1 to be carried out, the general conditions of the health insurance and their tariffs;
7. documents certifying the requirements for the members of the bodies of management under Art. 89;
8. document for the installed capital under Art. 87, paragraph 2;

9. declaration for the origin of the stock capital by the stock holders possessing stock over 10 000 levs at their face value;
10. document for paid licence fees;
11. structure of the company.

Art. 94. Within 1 month from submitting the documents under Art. 93 the Minister of Health shall make a proposal to the National Commission for Voluntary Health Insurance.

(2) Within 1 month from receipt of the proposal under paragraph 1 the National Commission for Voluntary Health Insurance shall take decision for the licensing of a company for voluntary health insurance.

Art. 95. The issuance of licence can be refused if:

1. the persons participating in the bodies of management of the company for voluntary health insurance do not meet the requirements of Art. 89;
2. the programme, the prognosis, the general conditions and the tariffs do not protect the interests of the insured or do not guarantee the fulfilment of the obligations;
3. other requirements of the law are not met;
4. the stock holding is provided by loans.

Art. 96. The issued licence to the company for voluntary health insurance can be withdrawn if:

1. conditions on the grounds of which it has been issued;
2. there are no programme, prognosis, general conditions and tariffs for the current budget year;
3. unlawfully refuses payment or pays by a delay of 3 months under the concluded insurance contracts;
4. activity is not carried out for a duration of 1 year from the issuance of the licence;
5. carries out other activity except the health insurance;
6. the voluntary principle of insurance and rendering medical care have not been complied with;
7. The annual balance has not been presented in time.

Art. 97. (1) Upon withdrawal of the licence the company for voluntary health insurance cannot conclude new insurance contracts, to continue the time of the existing ones or to expand payments on them.

(2) The withdrawal of the licence does not release the company for voluntary health insurance from its obligations under the concluded contracts.

Art. 98. The refusal to issue or the withdrawal of a licence shall be subject to appeal before the State Administrative Court within 14 days from the notification. The complaint shall be considered by the order of the Law for the administrative proceedings, as the consideration shall not stop the execution.

Art. 99. (1) The Ministry of Health shall keep a register of the companies to which licences are issued for voluntary health insurance.

(2) The contents of the register and the order of its keeping shall be determined by a decree of the Council of Ministers at the proposal of the Minister of Health.

Chapter IV. SPECIALISED HEALTH INSURANCE SUPERVISION

Art. 100. (1) The specialised supervision of the compulsory and voluntary health insurance shall be carried out by the Minister of Health.

(2) For providing the activity under paragraph 1 the Ministry of Health shall establish department "Specialised Health Insurance Supervision".

(3) The Council of Ministers shall determine the number of personnel of department "Specialised Health Insurance Supervision" at the proposal of the Minister of Health.

Art. 101. (1) Department "Specialised Health Insurance Supervision" shall:

1. control the lawfulness of the activities on the health insurance;
2. make proposals to the Minister of Health regarding the issuance or withdrawal of licences for voluntary health insurance;
3. keep the register under Art. 99, paragraph 1;
4. inform the respective court about the withdrawn licence of the company for voluntary health insurance;
5. analyse the entire activity on the compulsory and voluntary health insurance and prepare annual report for its status.

(2) The employees of department "Specialised Health Insurance Supervision" shall have the right to inspect NHIF, RHIF and the companies carrying out voluntary health insurance, for their activity. In carrying out the inspections they shall have the right of free access to the respective premises.

Art. 102. (1) The companies for voluntary health insurance shall present annually, at department "Specialised Health Insurance Supervision" a balance together with the necessary annexes for the condition of the type of health insurance for which they are licensed, within 3 months from expiration of the year of account.

(2) Department "Specialised Health Insurance Supervision" shall carry out current supervision over the activity of the companies for voluntary health insurance on the basis of the documents under paragraph 1, as well as by requiring current information about the activity at any time of the year of account.

(3) The companies for voluntary health insurance shall be obliged to present to the officials of department "Specialised Health Insurance Supervision" the documents, references, information and other carriers of information required by them, related to the voluntary health insurance.

Chapter V. ADMINISTRATIVE AND PUNITIVE PROVISIONS

Art. 103. (1) Official or employer, who does not present information, due under this law, or who presents untrue information about the insurance relations with NHIF shall be fined with 500 to 1 000 levs.
(2) For repeated and every next offence the fine shall be 2 000 levs.
(3) If the offence under paragraph 1 is made by an insured person the fine shall be 30 to 50 levs and in the cases under paragraph 2 - 150 levs.

Art. 104. (1) Official of employer or employer who does not pay the instalments for the insured persons, which are due, shall be fined with 500 to 1000 levs for each unpaid contribution.
(2) For repeated and for each next offence the fine shall be monthly 2000 levs for each unpaid contribution.

Art. 105. (1) The offences under Art. 103 and 104 shall be established by acts of the control bodies of the National Insurance Institute and NHIF.
(2) The penalty decrees shall be issued by the governor of the National Insurance Institute, by the Director of NHIF or by the Director of the respective Regional Health Insurance Fund and by the head of the respective division of the National Insurance Institute.

Art. 106. (1) For violation of the provisions of this law or of the normative acts for its implementation, except in the cases under Art. 103 and 104 a fine of 200 shall be imposed.
(2) The offences under paragraph 1 shall be established by acts issued by officials from department "Specialised Health Insurance Supervision" and the penalty decrees shall be issued by the Minister of Health.

Art. 107. The imposition of penalties under Art. 103 and 104 does not exclude the obligation to pay the due contributions together with the legal interest for the period.

Art. 108. (1) The issuance of acts, the issuance, the appeal and the fulfilment of the penalty decrees under this law shall be carried out according to the Law for the administrative offences and penalties.
(2) The imposed fines shall be deposited to the revenue of NHIF.

Art. 109. (1) Insured persons obliged to insure themselves and members of their families, who have not paid more than three due contributions, shall pay the medical care to the executives. When the insured person pays to the National Insurance Institute all due contributions his insurance rights shall be restored from the day of payment of the due contributions as the sums paid for the medical services shall not be restored.
(2) Failure to make insurance contributions for reasons beyond the control of the insured persons shall not deprive them of insurance rights. The sum paid for the medical service by the persons in these cases shall be subject to restoring.

Art. 110. For failure to appear for prophylactic examinations stipulated by NFC the insured shall lose the remaining rights for a period of 1 month.

Art. 111. The resources spent for treatment caused by premeditated damage to the own or other persons health, established by a court order, as well as for damaging the health as a result of alcohol abuse, shall be reimbursed to NHIF by the person who has caused it.

Additional provision

§ 1. In the context of this law:
1. "Assuring party" is the National Health Insurance Fund and the companies licensed for voluntary health insurance.
2. "Insured person" is an individual insured under the conditions and by the order of this law.
3. "Members of the family" are the spouse and the children under 18 years of age, and if they continue their education - until 26 years of age, and if they are incapacitated or permanently labour incapacitated - regardless of the age.
4. "Repeated" is an administrative offence made within 1 year from the enactment of the penalty decree by which the offender has been punished for the same offence.
5. "Insurance premium" is the sum that an individual or a corporate body shall pay under a contract with the company for voluntary health insurance.
6. "Person under proceedings for granting statute of refugee" is a foreign citizen or a person without citizenship who has requested statute of a refugee in the Republic of Bulgaria until the conclusion of the proceedings with enacted decision on his application.
7. "Medical care" represents a system of diagnostic, treatment, rehabilitation and prophylactic activities provided by medical specialists.
8. "Enterprise" are all corporate bodies, sole entrepreneurs and companies which are not legal entities carrying out trade activity.

Transitional and concluding provisions

§ 2. (1) The payment of the health insurance contributions under Art. 41 shall begin on July 1, 1999.

(2) The Minister of Health and the Minister of Finance can determine health establishments and surgeries where the payment shall be made on the basis of contracts before the introduction of the health insurance.

§ 3. (1) The fulfilment of the contracts between RHIF and the medical care executives on non-stationary level shall begin on July 1, 2000.

(2) The fulfilment of the contracts between RHIF and the hospitals shall begin on July 1, 2001.

(3) Until the commencement of the fulfilment of the contracts between the RHIF and the medical care executives under paragraph 1 and 2 the financing of the state and the municipal medical care and health establishments shall be carried out by the state and municipal budgets in a way applied till their transformation.

§ 4. The draft Law for the budget of NHIF for 2000 shall be presented at the Council of Ministers in 1999 within the period determined for presentation of the draft law for the state budget of the Republic of Bulgaria.

§ 5. Upon enactment of the law the Minister of Health shall begin the establishment of the structures and bodies stipulated by it. Upon constituting the bodies of NHIF the tasks on the establishment of the structures and carrying out the activities related to the compulsory health insurance shall be taken over by themselves.

§ 6. The Council of Ministers, the assemblies of the regions and the representative organisations of the employers and of the workers and employees shall, within 3 months from the enactment of the law, appoint its representatives in the Assembly of Representatives of NHIF.

§ 7. (1) Within 5 months from the enactment of the law the first meeting of the Assembly of Representatives of NHIF shall be held for election of Managing Board and Control Board.

(2) Within 1 month from constitution of the Assembly of Representatives regulations for the structure and activity of NHIF shall be adopted.

(3) Within 1 month from the constitution of the Managing Board a competition shall be held for appointment of director of NHIF.

§ 8. (1) Within 1 month from constitution of the bodies of NHIF the Managing Board shall open a procedure for preparation and negotiations under NFC.

(2) Within 3 months from the constitution of the bodies of NHIF the regulations stipulated by this law should be worked out and adopted.

§ 9. (1) The Council of Ministers, the regional governors and the municipalities shall, within 6 months from the enactment of the law, submit buildings and other material basis to the central management of NHIF and for RHIF.

(2) The Minister of Finance, at the proposal of the Minister of Health shall provide financial resources for the organisation of the process of establishing NHIF and RHIF.

§ 10. The Bulgarian National Bank shall open accounts of the companies for voluntary health insurance under Art. 3, paragraph 2 as the resources shall bear interest to the basic interest rate for the period.

§ 11. The receivables of NHIF for unpaid contributions or for delayed payment shall be collected with an interest which shall be equal to the basic interest rate for the period.

§ 12. The administrative support of NHIF and of RHIF for the periods under § 4 shall be for the account of the state budget.

§ 13. Item 7 is created in Art. 6, paragraph 1 of the Law for transformation and privatisation of state and municipal enterprises (promulgated in State Gazette, No 38 of 1992):

"7. For the National Health Insurance Fund - from the receipts under item 5 but not less than 50 percent of them."

§ 14. The following amendments and supplements are introduced to the Law for the national health (promulgated in State Gazette, No 88 of 1973):

1. In Art. 2, paragraph 1 is amended as follows:

"(1) Every Bulgarian citizen shall have the right to accessible medical care and health insurance stipulated by a law."

2. New Art. 3a is created:

"Art. 3a. The republican budget and the municipal budgets shall finance the activities of health care right to which have the citizens free of charge and related to:

1. emergency medical care;
2. stationary psychiatric care;
3. haemotransfusion;
4. compulsory immunisation and compulsory treatment under the Law for the National Health;
5. epidemiological and anti-epidemiological studies and activities;
6. health programmes and projects of national, regional and local importance;
7. state sanitary control;
8. investment expenses;
9. education, science and qualification;
10. construction for health purposes, basic repair, modernisation, improvement and reconstruction, as well as equipment over 10 million levs;
11. health administration;

12. national centres and institutes without direct treatment activity;
13. expensive treatment beyond the range of the compulsory health insurance by an order determined by the Minister of Health;
14. expenses related to the public health care;
15. expertise of the permanent labour disability and professional diseases."
3. The previous Art. 3a becomes Art. 3b.
4. The following amendments and supplements are introduced to Art. 4:
a) in paragraph 2, item, 1, after the words "medical care" is added "for the activities under Art. 3a";
b) paragraph 3 is revoked.
5. In Art. 4b, paragraph 1, after the words "the municipal budget" is added "revenue from the health insurance and payment in cash".
6. In Art. 25i paragraph 4 is created:
"(4) The regulations under paragraph 3 shall not apply for activities under contracts with the National Health Insurance Fund."
7. The following amendments and supplements are introduced to Art. 26:
a) paragraph 1 is amended as follows:
"(1) The persons under Art. 2, paragraph 1 shall have free choice and treatment by the physician and dentist for primary and specialised out-patient treatment on the territory of the respective Regional Health Insurance Fund.";
b) paragraph 2, 3, 4 and 5 are revoked.
8. In Art. 53, paragraph 2 the words "the order of Art. 26, paragraph 5" are replaced by "an order determined by the Minister of Health".
9. In Art. 55, paragraph 4 the words "and medical treatment" are deleted.
§ 15. In Art. 161, paragraph 3 of the Commercial Law the words "or insurance activity" are replaced by "insurance activity or activity on voluntary health insurance".
§ 16. In Art. 237, letter "c" of the Civil Procedural Code, after the words "the banks" is added "the Central Management of the National Health Insurance Fund and the Regional Health Insurance Funds".
§ 17. The following amendments are introduced to the Law for the defence and the armed forces:
1. In Art. 242, paragraph 1 and 2 are revoked.
2. In Art. 243, paragraph 1, 2 and 3 are revoked.
§ 18. In the Law for the Ministry of Internal Affairs (promulgated in State Gazette, No 122 of 1997, No 29 of 1998 - Decision No 3 of the Constitutional Court of 1998) Art. 224 is revoked.
§ 19. (1) Within 6 months from the enactment of the law the Council of Ministers, at the proposal of the Minister of Health shall adopt the normative acts related to its implementation.
(2) For the implementation of Art. 39 and Section V of the Law for the Council of Ministers ordinance shall be adopted at the proposal of the National Insurance Institute and NHIF.
§ 20. The fulfilment of the law is assigned to the Minister of Health, to the bodies of NHIF representing it and to the National Insurance Institute in the part for collection of health insurance contributions.

The law was adopted by the 38th National Assembly on June 4, 1998 and was affixed with the official seal of the National Assembly.